Ménière's Disease

A Beginner's 2-Week Step-by-Step Guide for Managing Meniere's Disease Through Diet, with Curated Recipes and a Sample Meal Plan

mf

copyright © 2021 Jeffrey Winzant

All rights reserved No part of this book may be reproduced, or stored in a retrieval system, or transmitted in any form or by any means, electronic, mechanical, photocopying, recording, or otherwise, without express written permission of the publisher.

Disclaimer

By reading this disclaimer, you are accepting the terms of the disclaimer in full. If you disagree with this disclaimer, please do not read the guide.

All of the content within this guide is provided for informational and educational purposes only, and should not be accepted as independent medical or other professional advice. The author is not a doctor, physician, nurse, mental health provider, or registered nutritionist/dietician. Therefore, using and reading this guide does not establish any form of a physician-patient relationship.

Always consult with a physician or another qualified health provider with any issues or questions you might have regarding any sort of medical condition. Do not ever disregard any qualified professional medical advice or delay seeking that advice because of anything you have read in this guide. The information in this guide is not intended to be any sort of medical advice and should not be used in lieu of any medical advice by a licensed and qualified medical professional.

The information in this guide has been compiled from a variety of known sources. However, the author cannot attest to or guarantee the accuracy of each source and thus should not be held liable for any errors or omissions.

You acknowledge that the publisher of this guide will not be held liable for any loss or damage of any kind incurred as a result of this guide or the reliance on any information provided within this guide. You acknowledge and agree that you assume all risk and responsibility for any action you undertake in response to the information in this guide.

Using this guide does not guarantee any particular result (e.g., weight loss or a cure). By reading this guide, you acknowledge that there are no guarantees to any specific outcome or results you can expect.

All product names, diet plans, or names used in this guide are for identification purposes only and are the property of their respective owners. The use of these names does not imply endorsement. All other trademarks cited herein are the property of their respective owners.

Where applicable, this guide is not intended to be a substitute for the original work of this diet plan and is, at most, a supplement to the original work for this diet plan and never a direct substitute. This guide is a personal expression of the facts of that diet plan.

Where applicable, persons shown in the cover images are stock photography models and the publisher has obtained the rights to use the images through license agreements with third-party stock image companies.

Table of Contents

Introduction	7
Overview	9
What triggers Ménière's disease?	9
Stages of Ménière's disease	10
How to Treat Ménière's Disease	12
Non-Surgical Treatments	12
Surgery	12
Tips to Manage the Disease	13
How to Approach a Low-Sodium Diet	14
The Different Types of Low Sodium Diets	16
Misconceptions about a Low Sodium Diet	16
Week 1–Plan to Reduce Sodium Intake	18
Step 1 – Determine your target intake	18
Step 2 – Determine your current intake	19
Step 3 – Purge the kitchen	19
Step 4 – Go shopping	19
Step 5 – Be mindful when eating out	19
Tips to Reduce Sodium Intake	20
Week 2–Diet Plan and Grocery Shopping	22
Grocery List	22
How to Read Nutrition Labels	23
Methods to Help with a Low-Sodium Meal Plan	24
Low Sodium When Eating with Others	26
7-Day Sample Meal Plan	26
Sample Recipes	29
Arugula and Mushroom Salad	30
Avocado, Cucumber, and Tomato Salad	31
Chicken Salad	32
Egg Salad with Avocados	33

Vegetable Broth	34
Avocado and Quinoa Salad	36
Salmon and Asparagus	37
Spinach, Feta, and Tomato Omelet	38
Seaweed Salad	39
Salad Medley	40
Quinoa-Based Asian Salad	42
Grenade Salad	43
Asian Zucchini Salad	44
Apple and Onion Soup	45
Mango Honey Green Smoothie	46
Turkey Sandwich	47
Conclusion	**48**
References and Helpful Links	**49**

Introduction

Around 45,500 people in the United States are diagnosed with Ménière's disease each year. 12 out of 1000 people are affected by the condition. If you think you are one of them, keep reading to find out how to treat Ménière's with your nutrition.

While it is a chronic disease, it is possible to treat it through a proper diet. However, it is crucial to get diagnosed by a doctor. A diagnosis can depend on several variables, such as two or more episodes of vertigo and a hearing test to determine the extent of loss of hearing.

Based on scientific studies, 6 out of 10 people can control their disease by changing their diet. Controlling the fluid in the inner ear with your diet can help control the symptoms. It involves eating regularly to manage the fluids in your body. As well as avoiding certain things like alcohol, chocolate, and caffeine that can worsen your headaches.

However, the most important part is keeping to a low sodium diet as sodium causes fluid retention and can aggravate your symptoms. Your diet should have two main goals; to stabilize your fluid levels and to avoid migraine trigger foods. This involves staying regular with your water intake throughout the day and avoiding foods and beverages with high salt and sugar content. With the proper dietary strategies, you can control fluctuations, headaches, and dizziness.

This may seem a lot to take in, which is why this guide is the perfect tool to teach you how to manage life with the disease and take it one step at a time.

In this guide, you will discover:

- The basics of Ménière's disease
- The different ways of treating Ménière's disease
- How to adopt a low sodium diet to treat Ménière's disease
- How to reduce your sodium intake
- Sample recipes for a low sodium diet

Overview

Ménière's disease is a condition that affects the inner ear. Since the ear is responsible for hearing and balance, the disease results in hearing loss, pressure deep inside the ear, tinnitus or buzzing in the ear, and episodes of dizziness known as vertigo. It usually affects only one ear but spreads to both ears with time, and while it is most likely to occur in a person's 40s or 50s, it can affect people at any age.

This might be the first time you are hearing about Ménière's disease, but do not worry. With the proper guidance, you can manage your symptoms and feel better instantly. Although it may take a while to get used to a new lifestyle, it is definitely worth it.

What triggers Ménière's disease?

There is no definite cause for this disease, but most scientists attribute it to changes in the fluid tubes of the inner ear. The build-up of fluid in the tubes causes these symptoms. Other underlying causes include allergies, autoimmune diseases, viral infections, or genetics.

Some of the most common symptoms include:

- Loss of balance
- Vertigo
- Tinnitus
- Headaches
- Nausea or Vomiting
- Decrease in hearing ability
- Sensitivity to noise

These symptoms usually come all at once and can last for up to 2-3 hours. The nature, duration, and severity of your symptoms are important in your diagnosis. During an attack, you may feel like the room is spinning and experience nausea and pressure in the ears. After an attack, you can experience mild hearing loss which will increase as the disease progresses.

Stages of Ménière's disease

The disease progresses in two stages. In the first stage, you may experience sudden bouts of dizziness with ringing or hearing loss. After the attack, you will most likely be exhausted and require rest.

In the later stage, you may experience fewer vertigo attacks, but your balance and hearing will deteriorate.

Here are some symptoms experienced after an attack:

- Anxiety, fear, irritation
- Appetite Fluctuation
- Difficulty concentrating
- Fatigue, sleepiness
- Lightheadedness, migraine
- Nausea, vomiting, motion sickness
- Heart palpitation, rapid pulse
- Sound sensitivity, trouble hearing
- Dizziness, difficulty walking, unsteadiness
- Vision difficulties, blurred vision

How to Treat Ménière's Disease

The disease does not have a cure, but there are several ways to treat it, prevent attacks and cope with the symptoms. Treatments usually vary depending on the severity of your attacks and the stage of your disease but here are the most common ones. Keep in mind that some of these treatments have to be prescribed by a doctor. Depending on the stage of the disease, your treatment will vary.

Non-Surgical Treatments

- Lifestyle changes - dietary alterations and stress management
- Motion sickness drugs to reduce nausea and dizziness
- Diuretics to reduce fluid retention
- Pressure pulse treatments to reduce pressure and vertigo

Surgery

If medical treatments are ineffective, surgery may be an option depending on the severity of your attacks. Some of the surgical options include:

- Endolymphatic sac decompression – to help control the buildup of fluid in the inner ear.
- Vestibular nerve section – to alter the balance mechanism in your inner ear.

Tips to Manage the Disease

Before you dive into surgical options, you may want to consider a less severe approach. Here are some tips to help you manage Ménière's disease:

- Make sure to take enough rest after an attack and avoid over-exerting yourself.
- Avoid potential triggers that can worsen your symptoms.
- Eat and drink water regularly throughout the day to manage your body fluids.
- Avoid smoking to decrease the severity of your symptoms.

In the next chapter, you'll find out how to approach a low-sodium diet to control Ménière's disease and further reduce your symptoms.

How to Approach a Low-Sodium Diet

Sodium is an essential mineral that has many functions in the body, such as controlling your body's fluid levels. Thus, a low-sodium diet and proper dietary strategies can help calm down your symptoms. The average American eats around 3,600 mg of sodium per day, so to adopt a low-sodium diet, you will need to make a few changes. You can create a nutrition plan by decreasing certain foods while supplementing others. It is also necessary to space out your meals and water intake evenly to stabilize the inner-ear fluid levels and avoid migraines.

The main aim is to avoid foods with a high salt or sugar content. This means focusing on whole foods with natural ingredients and limiting processed foods. You should aim for about 1,000 to 2,000 mg of sodium per day or, for reference, about 1/2 to 1 teaspoon of salt. Nonetheless, it might be appropriate to consult your doctor to determine your target intake.

When starting a low-sodium diet, you want to educate yourself about the foods you usually eat as much as possible. For example, many processed foods contain monosodium glutamate or MSG which contains large amounts of sodium. Store-bought foods such as curated meats, dehydrated soups, sauces and marinades, canned foods, and salted snacks also have a large amount of sodium.

It helps to read the food nutrition labels of each product to find out the sodium content. One helpful tip is to know that the ingredients listed first on the label are usually in higher content within the food.

To approach a low-sodium diet, we'll cover how to reduce your sodium intake in week one, and in week two, we'll cover how you should eat and some sample recipes to help you out.

Another helpful strategy is to use a food tracker app. Although these apps are for tracking calories and macros, you can use them to track your sodium levels and find out how much sodium each meal has. This makes it easier for you to track your sodium intake in the first few weeks until you get the hang of it. With time you will be able to eat intuitively, without needing to track.

The Different Types of Low Sodium Diets

General Low-Sodium Diet

Limiting your sodium intake without any clear target to hit. Your doctor might suggest this if you are just starting or you are in the early stages of the disease.

3,000 mg-Sodium Diet

This diet involves limiting your sodium intake below 3,000 mg, it is not as severe. Your doctor should help advise you whether this is the one for you.

2,000 mg-Sodium Diet

On this diet, you should limit yourself to 2,000 mg of sodium or less per day. The most common and advised option for Ménière's disease.

Misconceptions about a Low Sodium Diet

Sea salt is an alternative – regardless of the source, sodium is still sodium and even sea salt will increase your sodium intake.

Sodium only comes from salt – even whole foods contain some sodium which is why it is advised not to add salt to your cooking.

Sodium is bad for you – just because you need a low-sodium diet to help manage your symptoms does not mean that sodium is bad for you. You still need the mineral for normal cell and muscle function.

Week 1–Plan to Reduce Sodium Intake

In the first week, you need to focus on reducing your sodium intake to at least below 2000mg. We've broken down the guide into two weeks to make it easier for you to adapt to this new lifestyle. By taking it step-by-step, you will be more equipped to sustain this new regimen.

You might find it difficult to adapt to a low-sodium diet at first because salt is a key seasoning in almost every meal. Thus, you need to be selective about what you eat in relation to that and be more mindful of sodium in other foods. Here are a few methods and tips to help you stick to a low-sodium diet:

Step 1 – Determine your target intake

Before you dive headfirst into the diet, you need to determine how much sodium you are allowed to have. This will vary for every person, some may have a more severe limit than others.

Step 2 – Determine your current intake

It might be helpful to find out your current sodium intake beforehand. You can download a sodium-tracking app to assess how much sodium you consume during a normal day or you can use a template like the one made by the American Heart Association.

Step 3 – Purge the kitchen

So on day one, you want to get rid of the salty snacks and products that are high in sodium. If you don't see it, you will not reach for it. If you live with other people, then make sure that you cannot access these high-sodium foods or designate a place in the kitchen that you are not exposed to.

Step 4 – Go shopping

Now that you've purged your space of the foods that are harmful to your diet, you want to stock up on the things you can have. Things like fresh produce, low-sodium alternatives, and unsalted snacks are great options. Often health food stores have great options for low-sodium cheeses, condiments, and snacks.

Step 5 – Be mindful when eating out

When you're eating out, it may be more challenging to control your sodium intake, so it's best to be selective and opt for lower sodium options as much as possible. Avoid as many processed foods as you can; foods such as bacon, cheese, curated meats, and sauces are high in sodium. With a bit of planning, you can enjoy eating out. It's useful to check out the menu of the restaurant beforehand, and you can also ask them not to add extra salt to your meal.

Tips to Reduce Sodium Intake

- Add less salt to your food when cooking or try to omit it since 1 tablespoon of salt contains about 2,300 mg of sodium. Instead, add plenty of herbs and seasonings like garlic, lemon, and pepper.
- Beware of condiments and sauces as they usually contain a lot of salt. Find substitutes instead. For example, replace soy sauce with coconut aminos. The former holds 280 mg sodium per 5ml, while coconut aminos contain only 90 mg.
- Avoid fast foods as they are usually packed with salt. As well as frozen meals, processed meats like bacon, and pickled foods.
- Plant-based foods usually contain less sodium than animal-based foods like meat and dairy. So it's beneficial to pack in as many vegetables and greens as you can into your diet.
- Use lemon juice and olive oil to replace the usual salad dressings. It is better to make your dips, sauces, and marinades to control your sodium intake.

- Be mindful of sodium substitutes and consult your doctor to know about any potential nutrient interactions.
- Remember that even if it isn't salty, it can contain high amounts of sodium. Sodium is often used as a preservative and to help balance out the taste in foods such as bread and even desserts.
- Spread out your sodium intake throughout the day. A higher sodium meal, even if you remain below your limit, can trigger your symptoms.
- Cut back on the sodium gradually. Going all in may shock you at first, and it will be difficult to maintain the diet. It's best to take the first week slowly decreasing the amount of sodium you are having.
- Keep a diary to track your progress and journal your mood and symptoms with the diet. This is a useful tip to help assess how successful the changes in your diet are and how you feel in each step.
- Be careful of medications that contain sodium. Sodium is a common ingredient in antacids, painkillers, and laxatives, so make sure to consult your doctor before taking any.
- Avoid soft water because it often has added sodium, and check the labels of any bottled water.

Week 2–Diet Plan and Grocery Shopping

Now that you know what foods to avoid, let's focus on the foods you can have. Week 2 centers around helping you with your low-sodium meal plan. Let's start with a sample grocery list to help you set your meal plan for success.

Grocery List

- Frozen and fresh vegetables and fruits
- Sweet potatoes / unsalted chickpeas / cabbage / broccoli
- Cucumber / green beans / green peppers / lettuce
- Fresh or dried herbs without salt
- Snacks that are unsalted, low in sodium, or sodium-free–unsalted nuts and popcorn, dark chocolate
- Fresh or frozen meats that have not been pre-marinated or seasoned
- Eggs and low-sodium cheeses and dairy products
- Dry beans and grains that are not canned
- Bread without salted coatings
- Most carbs are safe; oats, quinoa, pasta, rice, etc

- Vegetable oils and unsalted butter are good

Remember to check the ingredient labels and compare products to find the ones lower in sodium. Be aware that low sodium labels can also be misleading. The FDA has some leeway with these labels, and it only means that the food is relatively lower in sodium. To be safe, you want to avoid processed foods as much as possible and concentrate on whole foods. A good rule of thumb is if there are too many ingredients in one product, it is best to avoid it. It's also handy to be mindful of the type of cuisine you are eating; for example, many Asian sauces and food items contain a lot of salt.

To keep track of your sodium intake, you can keep a journal or use a food app. Track throughout the day to make sure you are evenly spreading out your consumption.

How to Read Nutrition Labels

- Sodium-free usually means less than 5 mg of sodium per serving.
- Low sodium signifies 149 mg of sodium or less per serving.
- Reduced sodium is equal to 25% less sodium compared to the original version of the product.
- Unsalted means that salt is not added during processing but the product is not necessarily sodium-free.

Methods to Help with a Low-Sodium Meal Plan

Step 1: Meal Plan

One helpful habit can be to start meal planning; this will make it easier to plan your meals and sodium intake in advance. If your meals are already planned and made beforehand, you are less likely to reach for quick meals that might compromise your low-sodium diet.

Prepping your meals means that you can control every compartment that goes into the meal and understand how it all adds up. When cooking, you want to calculate the sodium content in each ingredient and avoid using additional salt.

This may seem challenging at first, especially if you enjoy salty foods, your new diet may seem bland. However, with time you will get used to eating without added salt, and it doesn't mean your food has to be completely unseasoned. Use herbs and spices to bring up the dish and replace salt with lemon juice or anything acidic.

Designate a day and take a few hours to prepare your meals for the next few days or even the week. You can either prep full meals or prep various components that you can build up into different meals. One day of meal prep can be cooking a small batch of chicken breasts or any other protein, prepping two types of carbs for the week, and veggies. However, when it comes to greens, it is best to keep them fresh so that you can add a drizzle of lemon and omit the salt.

Step 2: Experiment with Your Cooking

To adapt to a low-sodium diet, it's best to make your own seasoning, marinades, and dips. Experiment with different spices and find combinations you like, for example, something simple like garlic and thyme can brighten up the dish. You can also experiment with baking and snacks like homemade granola instead of buying it.

Step 3: Find Alternatives to the Foods You Love

Just because you are on a low-sodium diet, it doesn't mean you have to sacrifice the meals you enjoy. You can buy low-sodium alternatives or make your own version at home. For example, instead of buying fries, you can make your own in the oven or air fryer without salt or added seasoning.

Step 4: Remember to Keep It Simple

It's best to keep your meals simple at first to keep track of your sodium intake. If you stick to basic meal components; good carbs, protein, fats, and greens, you'll effectively meet your goals. If you are adding too many ingredients to one dish, you might find the sodium levels going up. So stick to whole, non-processed ingredients when cooking.

Low Sodium When Eating with Others

If you are not living alone and you have to cook for others or eat what they are cooking, adopting a low-sodium diet may become more challenging than it is.

But if that's the case, you can either cook your meal apart, or you can make everything low sodium and allow the others to add their salt to taste after.

Now that you know how to get started, let's look at what a 7-day meal plan would look like for you!

7-Day Sample Meal Plan

Day 1

- Breakfast - Berry oatmeal
- Lunch - Chicken salad
- Snack - Unsalted nuts & dried fruit
- Dinner - Roasted salmon with asparagus

Day 2

- Breakfast - Banana Smoothie
- Lunch - Pasta salad
- Snack - Chia pudding
- Dinner - Veggie stuffed chicken breasts

Day 3

- Breakfast - Spinach omelet

- Lunch - Quinoa salad
- Snack - Mango smoothie
- Dinner - One-pan veggie and beef stir-fry

Day 4

- Breakfast - Toast with unsalted butter and poached eggs
- Lunch - One-pot lemon chicken and rice
- Snack - Greek yogurt with fruit
- Dinner - Turkey with roasted potatoes

Day 5

- Breakfast - Fresh fruit salad and omelet
- Lunch - Avocado and tomato salad
- Snack - Unsalted popcorn
- Dinner - Steak with vegetable medley

Day 6

- Breakfast - Homemade granola and yogurt
- Lunch - Beet, orange, and feta salad
- Snack - Homemade hummus dip and carrots
- Dinner - Chicken, mushrooms, and rice

Day 7

- Breakfast - Overnight oats
- Lunch - Veggie sandwich
- Snack - Dark chocolate and strawberries

- Dinner - Spicy baked fish with quinoa

Now that you've seen what a low-sodium meal plan can look like, rest assured that your diet doesn't have to be plain or boring. In the next chapter, you can take a look at a few sample recipes that you can incorporate into your diet. The best part is that you can adapt them to your tastes and switch out the carbs, veggies, or proteins.

Sample Recipes

Arugula and Mushroom Salad

Ingredients:

- 5 oz. arugula washed
- 1 lb. fresh mushrooms
- 1/4 tsp. shoyu
- 1/2 red onion
- 1 tbsp. olive oil
- 1 tbsp. mirin

For tofu cheese:

- 1/8 cup umeboshi vinegar
- 1/2 firm tofu

Instructions:

1. In a bowl, add the rinsed tofu. Crumble and pour in vinegar.
2. In a separate bowl add shoyu, red onions, salt, olive oil, and mirin. 3. Mix to combine.
3. Add in the arugula and toss to combine with the dressing.
4. Serve and enjoy.

Avocado, Cucumber, and Tomato Salad

Ingredients:

- 1/4 cup extra-virgin olive oil
- 1 pc. lemon, juiced
- 1/4 tsp. cumin, ground
- salt, to taste
- freshly ground black pepper, to taste
- 3 medium avocados, cubed
- 1-pint cherry tomatoes, halved
- 1 small cucumber, sliced into half-moons
- 1/3 cup corn
- 2 tbsp. cilantro, chopped

Instructions:

1. Combine avocados, cilantro, corn, cucumber, jalapeño, and tomatoes in a large bowl.
2. In a separate small container, whisk together lemon juice, cumin, and oil to make the salad dressing.
3. Season the dressing with salt and pepper.
4. Toss the salad gently while adding the dressing.
5. Serve immediately.

Chicken Salad

Ingredients:

- 1 small can of premium chunk chicken breast packed in water
- 1 stalk celery, large, finely chopped
- 1/4 cup reduced-fat mayonnaise
- 4 romaine leaves or red leaf lettuce, washed and trimmed
- 8 pcs. cherry tomatoes or 1 ripe tomato, quartered
- 1 cucumber, small and sliced thinly

Instructions:

1. Drain canned chicken and transfer to a bowl.
2. Put in celery and mayonnaise.
3. Mix lightly. Don't crush the chicken.
4. In a separate shallow bowl, place the lettuce neatly.
5. Add the chicken salad in the middle
6. Add tomatoes and cucumber slices to the plate.
7. Refrigerate before serving, cover with plastic wrap.

Egg Salad with Avocados

Ingredients:

- 3 medium-sized avocados
- 6 eggs, large and hard-boiled
- 1/3 red onion, medium size
- 3 celery ribs
- 4 tbsps. mayonnaise
- 2 tbsps. freshly squeezed lime juice
- 2 tsp. brown mustard
- 1/2 tsp. cumin powder
- 1 tsp. hot sauce
- salt
- pepper

Instructions:

1. Chop the eggs, celery, and onion.
2. Set aside the avocados, then combine the rest of the ingredients.
3. Slice the avocado in half to take out the pit.
4. Stuff the avocado by spooning the egg salad on its cave.
5. Serve and enjoy.

Vegetable Broth

Ingredients:

- 1 tbsp. oil
- 2 leeks, sliced
- 2 carrots, sliced
- 2 ribs celery
- 1/4 tsp. salt
- 8 cups water

To make the soup:

- 1 tbsp. oil
- 2 cups potatoes, diced
- 1 cup mushrooms, diced
- 1-1/2 cups cauliflower, diced
- 1 cup onion, diced
- 1 cup celery, diced
- 1 cup carrot, diced
- 1-1/2 cups red beans, cooked
- 2 sprigs rosemary
- 4 sprigs thyme
- 2 cups spinach

Instructions:

1. To a pot on medium heat, add oil and leeks.
2. Cook for about three minutes or until they start to soften up.

3. Add carrots and top a few celery stalks with leaves.
4. Cover with water.
5. Add salt. Bring to a simmer and cook until carrots are very tender but not mushy.
6. Turn off the heat and let it cool down a little.
7. When the broth has cooled down, strain out the veggies.
8. Remove carrots and set them aside.
9. Squeeze most of the liquid out of the leeks and celery.

To cook the soup:

1. Add carrots to some of the broth and blend.
2. With a pot on medium heat, add oil, onions, raw carrots, and celery. Cook until onions are translucent, approximately 3 to 5 minutes.
3. Add broth, potatoes, and herbs.
4. Bring to a simmer and cook for 10 minutes.
5. Add cauliflower and red beans.
6. Simmer for another 5 minutes.
7. Add the package of frozen green beans and cook until the potatoes and cauliflower are tender, approximately for another 5 minutes.
8. At the end of cooking, add spinach.
9. Serve warm.

Avocado and Quinoa Salad

Ingredients:

- 4 avocados cut into pieces
- 1 cup of quinoa
- 400 grams of chickpeas
- 30 grams of fresh parsley

Instructions:

1. In a pot, boil quinoa with 2 cups of water.
2. Reduce heat to a simmer, cover, and cook for 12 minutes until water is evaporated.
3. Fluff with a fork until grains are swollen and glassy.
4. Toss all the ingredients together.
5. Season with sea salt and black pepper.
6. Serve warm with lemon wedges and olive oil.

Salmon and Asparagus

Ingredients:

- 2 salmon filets
- 14-oz. young potatoes
- 8 asparagus spears, trimmed and halved
- 2 handfuls cherry tomatoes
- 1 handful basil leaves
- 2 tbsp. extra-virgin olive oil
- 1 tbsp. balsamic vinegar

Instructions:

1. Heat oven to 428°F.
2. Arrange potatoes into a baking dish.
3. Drizzle potatoes with extra-virgin olive oil.
4. Roast potatoes until they have turned golden brown.
5. Place asparagus into the baking dish together with the potatoes.
6. Roast in the oven for 15 minutes.
7. Arrange cherry tomatoes and salmon among the vegetables.
8. Drizzle with balsamic vinegar and the remaining olive oil.
9. Roast until the salmon is cooked.
10. Throw in basil leaves before transferring everything to a serving dish.
11. Serve while hot.

Spinach, Feta, and Tomato Omelet

Ingredients:

- cooking spray
- 1/4 cup Roma tomatoes, chopped
- 3/4 cup Egg Beaters Liquid Egg Whites
- 2 tbsp. fat reduced feta cheese, crumbled
- 1/8 tsp. ground black pepper
- 1/4 cup baby spinach leaves, chopped

Instructions:

1. Spray small amounts of cooking spray in a nonstick skillet. Heat over medium heat.
2. Cook the Egg Beaters in the skillet, and season with pepper. Cook for 2 minutes.
3. Lift the edges to cook the other side of the egg. Cook for 3 more minutes.
4. Top half of the omelet with tomatoes, spinach, and feta cheese. Fold the other half of the omelet over the filling.
5. Serve.

Seaweed Salad

Ingredients:

- 4 tsp. fish sauce
- 2 oz. dried seaweed such as wakame, arame, dulse, or agar
- 2 green onions, finely chopped
- 1 tsp. fresh ginger juice
- 2 tbsp. coconut water vinegar
- 2 tsp. honey
- 2 cups cucumber, finely sliced
- 1/4 cup fresh lemon juice
- 2 cups daikon radish or Japanese turnip, finely sliced

Instructions:

1. Mix together the honey, coconut water vinegar, lemon juice, fish sauce, and ginger juice to create a salad dressing.
2. Immerse the seaweed in cold water for at least 5 minutes, or until it is adequately soft.
3. Rinse and drain after. Chop if the pieces are too big.
4. Combine the rehydrated seaweed with turnips, radish, cucumber, and dressing.
5. Top with green onions as a garnish.
6. Serve and enjoy.

Salad Medley

Ingredients:

- 4 artichokes, halved
- 1/2 avocado, sliced into thin wedges
- 1/2 red, yellow, or green bell pepper, thinly sliced
- 1/4 squash, thinly sliced
- 1/2 zucchini, thinly sliced
- 1/2 red, yellow, or green onion, thinly sliced
- 1 cup mushrooms, thinly sliced
- 1 cup broccoli
- 1/4 cup broccoli sprouts
- 1 cup cauliflower
- 1 cup spinach
- 1 cup kale
- 1 bunch leeks, chopped
- 1/4 cup raw sunflower seeds, sprouted
- 1/4 cup raw almonds, sprouted
- 1/4 cup garbanzo beans, sprouted
- 1/4 cup mung beans, sprouted
- 1/4 cup red or green lentils, sprouted
- 1/4 cup purple cabbage, shredded
- 2 tbsp. extra-virgin olive oil

Instructions:

1. Steam vegetables in a saucepan with 1-inch water for 5 to 10 minutes.

2. Transfer steamed vegetables into a serving bowl.
3. Drizzle with extra-virgin olive oil.
4. Toss the vegetables.
5. Serve immediately.

Quinoa-Based Asian Salad

Ingredients:

- 2 cups uncooked quinoa
- 4 cups vegetable broth
- 1 cup edamame
- 1/4 cup green onion, chopped
- 1-1/2 tsp. fresh mint, chopped
- 1/2 cup carrot, chopped
- 1/8 tsp. pepper flakes
- 1/2 tsp. orange zest, grated
- 2 tbsp. fresh Thai basil, chopped
- juice from half an orange
- 1 tsp. sesame seeds
- 1 tsp. sesame oil
- 1 tbsp. olive oil
- 1/8 tsp. black pepper

Instructions:

1. Mix the broth and quinoa in a pan.
2. Set the stove to high. Place the pan.
3. Let the mixture heat up for 12 to 14 minutes.
4. After heating, cover the pan and wait for 4 minutes.
5. Place the mixture in a separate container. Add in the rest of the ingredients.
6. Let it cool down before serving.

Grenade Salad

Ingredients:

- 4 cups arugula
- 1 large avocado
- 1/2 cup sliced fennel
- 1/2 cup sliced Anjou pears
- /4 cup pomegranate seeds

Instructions:

1. Mix all the ingredients except for the pomegranate seeds.
2. After mixing well, add the seeds. Mix again.
3. Serve with any type of desired dressing.

Asian Zucchini Salad

Ingredients:

- 1 medium zucchini, sliced thinly into spirals
- 1/3 cup rice vinegar
- 3/4 cup avocado oil
- 1 cup sunflower seeds, shells removed
- 1 lb. cabbage, shredded
- 1 tsp. stevia drops
- 1 cup almonds, sliced

Instructions:

1. Cut the zucchini spirals into smaller parts. Set aside.
2. Put almonds, sunflower seeds, and cabbage in a large bowl. Combine the ingredients well.
3. Add zucchini to the mixture.
4. In a small bowl, mix vinegar, stevia, and oil using a whisk or fork.
5. Pour the vinegar mixture all over the zucchini mixture. Toss well. Make sure everything is covered with the dressing.
6. Refrigerate for 2 hours before serving.

Apple and Onion Soup

Ingredients:

- 3 organic apples, diced
- 2 medium yellow onions, sliced
- 6 cups vegetable broth
- 1 small leek, chopped
- 1 tbsp. avocado oil
- 1/2 tbsp. fresh rosemary, chopped
- 1/2 tbsp. fresh thyme

Instructions:

1. Place the saucepan over medium heat.
2. Pour the avocado oil into the saucepan.
3. Add the onion slices. Sauté until the color has turned golden.
4. Pour in the vegetable broth.
5. Bring to a boil over medium heat.
6. Add the diced apples.
7. Reduce the heat to the medium-low setting.
8. Simmer for 10 minutes.
9. Serve immediately.

Mango Honey Green Smoothie

Ingredients:

- 2 pcs. bananas
- a handful of large spinach
- 1 pc. mango, sliced
- 1 tbsp. honey
- 3-4 pcs. ice cubes

Instructions:

1. Put all the ingredients in a blender.
2. Blend until smooth.
3. Serve and enjoy.

Turkey Sandwich

Ingredients:

- 3 oz. roasted turkey, sliced
- 2 oz. whole wheat pita bread
- a few pcs. romaine lettuce leaves
- 1 tsp. mustard
- 2 slices tomato
- 1/2 cup grapes, cut in half

Instructions:

1. Cut pita bread in half, fully opening the pocket in the middle.
2. Layer the ingredients inside each pita bread slice.
3. Briefly heat in the microwave oven or on a pan if desired.
4. Serve and enjoy while warm.

Conclusion

There you have it! Our guide to managing the symptoms of Ménière's disease. It's no secret that Ménière's is a tedious disease to keep under control, but implementing all of these methods could make a huge difference in your health.

While the disease can be unpredictable, living with Ménière's disease is possible. We hope you find the right methods for your lifestyle. Remember that if you find it stressful or overwhelming, it is always a good idea to join a support group or talk to your doctor about getting help.

Thank you again for getting this guide.

If you found this guide helpful, please take the time to share your thoughts and post a review. It'd be greatly appreciated!

Thank you and good luck!

References and Helpful Links

Diet for Meniere's disease. (n.d.). Retrieved December 11, 2022, from https://dizziness-and-balance.com/disorders/menieres/treatment/diet.html

Dietary recommendations for managing dizziness. (n.d.). Vestibular Disorders Association. Retrieved December 11, 2022, from https://vestibular.org/article/coping-support/living-with-a-vestibular-disorder/dietary-considerations/

Eating well with Meniere's disease. (n.d.). Retrieved December 11, 2022, from https://muschealth.org/medical-services/ent/otology/vertigo/eating-well

Guidelines for a low sodium diet. (n.d.). Ucsfhealth.Org. Retrieved December 11, 2022, from https://www.ucsfhealth.org/education/guidelines%20for%20a%20low%20sodium%20diet

How I manage my Meniere's symptoms with a low sodium diet. (n.d.). Healthy Hearing. Retrieved December 11, 2022, from https://www.healthyhearing.com/report/53004-Managing-menieres-symptoms-with-a-low-sodium-diet

Low-sodium diet: Benefits, food lists, risks and more. (2018, December 10). Healthline. https://www.healthline.com/nutrition/low-sodium-diet

Meniere disease - self-care: MedlinePlus Medical Encyclopedia. (n.d.). Retrieved December 11, 2022, from https://medlineplus.gov/ency/patientinstructions/000709.htm

Meniere's disease: Symptoms, causes, treatments, and more. (2012, August 15). Healthline. https://www.healthline.com/health/menieres-disease

Meniere's disease: Treatment, symptoms, stages, and diet. (2020, April 14). https://www.medicalnewstoday.com/articles/163888

Ménière's disease. (2017, October 19). Nhs.Uk. https://www.nhs.uk/conditions/menieres-disease/

Services, D. of H. & H. (n.d.). Ears—Meniere's disease. Retrieved December 11, 2022, from http://www.betterhealth.vic.gov.au/health/conditionsandtreatments/ears-menieres-disease

What is ménière's disease? — Diagnosis and treatment. (n.d.). NIDCD. Retrieved December 11, 2022, from https://www.nidcd.nih.gov/health/menieres-disease

www.ingramcontent.com/pod-product-compliance
Lightning Source LLC
LaVergne TN
LVHW051925060526
838201LV00062B/4690